Notes on Orthopaedic Nursing

Jane T. Webb SRN ONC
Senior Nurse, Paediatric Orthopaedics, Royal National Orthopaedic
Hospital, Stanmore, Middlesex

Foreword by
Michael A. Edgar MChir FRCS
Consultant Orthopaedic Surgeon, Royal National Orthopaedic Hospital,
Stanmore, Middlesex

SECOND EDITION

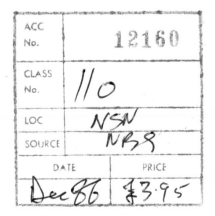

CHURCHILL LIVINGSTONE
EDINBURGH LONDON MELBOURNE AND NEW YORK 1985

CHURCHILL LIVINGSTONE
Medical Division of Longman Group Limited

Distributed in the United States of America by
Churchill Livingstone Inc., 1560 Broadway, New York,
N.Y. 10036, and by associated companies, branches,
and representatives throughout the world.

First edition 1977
Second edition 1985

ISBN 0 443 03162 2

British Library Cataloguing in Publication Data
Webb, Jane T.
    Notes on orthopaedic nursing. — 2nd ed.
    1. Orthopedic nursing
    I. Title
    610.73'677   RD753

Library of Congress Cataloging in Publication Data
Webb, Jane T.
    Notes on orthopaedic nursing.
    (Churchill Livingstone nursing notes)
    Bibliography: p.
    Includes index.
    1. Orthopedic nursing — Outlines, syllabi, etc.
I. Title. II. Series. [DNLM: 1. Orthopedics —
nursing — outlines. WY 18 W366n]
RD753.W37   1985   610.73   84–12058

Printed in Singapore by
Selector Printing Co (Pte) Ltd

Foreword

Jane Webb's excellent little book has already become a popular and established work in its field as a result of the first edition, where the foreword was written by the late Charles Manning. In writing the foreword to the second edition, therefore, it is a double honour for me to be associated with two people who have contributed so much to orthopaedics, and especially to its practice at the Royal National Orthopaedic Hospital, Stanmore.

The following pages are not meant to be comprehensive for this is the role of the bulky textbook. In this slender tome the essential features of orthopaedics and trauma are covered with precision, balance and clarity. It is difficult to be brief and yet to maintain an attractive and readable style. The author must be complimented for having achieved this combination so well.

The size of the book is ideal for the pocket, handbag or briefcase according to the occasion, be it the ward or the bus. It is not designed for the bookshelf; it is meant to be used. The first edition certainly was, and undoubtedly the second will be also.

Middlesex, 1985   M.A.E.

Preface

The idea behind this book is to present the orthopaedic syllabus in a brief synoptic form. Quick reference is an advantage throughout training and particularly whilst revising for examinations.

It is hoped that the information will be of use, not only to nurses studying for their Orthopaedic Nursing Certificate, but also to students, qualified nurses, physiotherapists and other paramedical staff who wish to know more about orthopaedics.

Nurses and physiotherapists all receive a basic training in anatomy and physiology which is not included in this small book, but I hope they may use it in connection with their larger tomes. A suggested reading list to be used in conjunction with this book may be found on page 95.

I would like to thank my mother for all her help typing the script and all my friends at work for their encouragement.

Middlesex, 1977   J. T. W.

Second edition

Orthopaedic nursing never stands still. I have attempted to up-date this book, maintaining the note form.

Many more diagrams have been included, which I hope will clarify the text. Larger sections are included on children's topics and rheumatological conditions.

Middlesex, 1985   J. T. W.

Contents

Introduction

Over the past two decades the type of work done in ortho-paedic units and wards has changed considerably. Trauma, of course, continues but with modern treatments and trends the patient is out of hospital far quicker. Since the introduction of the compulsory use of seat belts, the number of facial and associated injuries has been reduced. The introduction of arthroscopes has meant that diagnoses may be confirmed more accurately, and in fact some operations such as a menisectomy can now be performed through an arthroscope.

Despite the fact that treatments now take less time, the waiting lists for orthopaedic operations still lengthen – perhaps because far more is now on offer to patients. Replacement surgery is becoming almost commonplace. With the general population now living much longer, orthopaedics have a very important part to play in keeping the elderly patient mobile, pain-free and independent. Tumours in bones used to mean an early death, particularly for children and young adults, but the combination of chemotherapy with custom-made prostheses for the patient has changed the outlook considerably.

New cases of poliomyelitis are rarely seen these days; the orthopaedic care required is normally for the patient who developed the disease during the outbreaks thirty to forty years ago, and now presents with joint problems, due often to the unequal strain that has been put on to the sound joint. Tuberculosis has not disappeared completely, but with modern-day testing and immunisation it is more commonly seen in foreign people who have settled in this country or who are studying here.

Rehabilitation is now a very important topic in any orthopaedic syllabus. As with most orthopaedic conditions, teamwork in a rehabilitation unit is extremely important. Independence for the individual is greatly desired and this must be worked for and attained if at all possible. Nursing the rehabilitating patient is particularly difficult – having to stand by and watch someone struggle to achieve a goal is far more stressful than giving the helping hand, but the latter does nothing to help the patient.

Perhaps over the next twenty years things will develop to such an extent that it may be possible to repair the spinal cord, enabling paraplegic patients to walk again; perhaps the reason for idiopathic conditions such as scoliosis will be discovered; and if the cause of rheumatoid arthritis cannot be found, perhaps cures will be discovered that prevent the deterioration in joints. Osteoarthritis I fear will always be with us, but the growing interest in diets and keep-fit programmes can only lead to a healthier population. We already have replacement prostheses for the hip, knee, shoulder, elbow and finger joints, but no doubt others will be added to this list before long.

1

Orthopaedic conditions

The following chapter outlines the main conditions in orthopaedics and common types of surgery performed. Individual conditions will be found under the relevant chapter.

Tuberculosis

Incidence of disease is decreasing. Tuberculous bacillus may be either human or bovine. It reaches bone through blood stream from other foci e.g. intestinal tract or lungs. Bacillus may infect bone or synovial membrane. Causes inflammatory reaction followed by necrosis of bone and tissue.

Larger joints more commonly affected, also spine. Synovial membrane becomes thickened and inflamed. Articular cartilage destroyed and underlying bone eroded. Cold abscesses may form and track down muscles to skin surface: may rupture and form sinus.

Patient is usually child or young adult. Complains of pain, swelling and lack of movement in joint. Joint often warm and surrounding muscles wasted. Erythrocyte sedimentation rate raised. Mantoux test positive. Joint aspiration may confirm diagnosis. Careful check necessary to exclude other tuberculous foci.

Treatment. Rest, good diet, fresh air and anti-tuberculous drugs, e.g. rifampicin and isoniazid which are usually given with either ethambutol, streptomycin or pyrazinamide. A combination of three drugs is necessary and they must be continued for a minimum of six months. Affected joint or spine rested in bed. Plaster splintage may be helpful.

Abscesses drained if necessary. When disease quiescent erythrocyte sedimentation rate will drop. Physiotherapy commenced on affected joint until movement restored. If particular cartilage has been destroyed joint will be painful and non-functioning. Arthrodesis of joint in optimum position of function may be necessary.

Infective arthritis

Infection of joint by bacteria. May enter joint from bloodstream, externally from wound or extend from focus of osteomyelitis already in body. Any age group affected. Onset may be acute or insidious. Patient ill and pyrexial; affected joint hot and swollen due to effusion in joint and thickening of synovial membrane. X-rays show no change at start of disease. White cell count and erythrocyte sedimentation rate both raised.

Treatment. Bed rest and good diet. Causative organism identified if possible by culture of joint aspirate. Broad-spectrum antibiotics may be commenced before sensitivity reports available. Appropriate antibiotics given for minimum of three months. Joint rested in plaster, on traction or bed rest. Excessive fluid may be aspirated to relieve tension in joint. Antibiotics may be injected locally into joint. When disease quiescent, physiotherapy commenced to restore joint movement. If joint damage has been severe and recovery impossible, arthrodesis of joint at later date will render it painfree.

Rheumatoid arthritis

Chronic systemic disease affecting many joints. Occurs mainly in women between 25 and 45 years. Similar disease affecting children is Still's disease. Cause unknown. Small joints affected first. Onset gradual. Synovial membrane inflamed causing swelling of joint, capsule and tissues, effusion into joint and thinning of adjacent bone. All cause pain and stiffness. Erythrocyte sedimentation rate will be raised and haemoglobin often lowered. Rheumatoid factor will be positive. Synovial biopsy performed to exclude infection. See Chapter 8.

Treatment. Bed rest in acute stages, with splints or plaster casts to support joints. Analgesic and anti-inflammatory drugs given. Passive physiotherapy followed by active use of joints as pain lessens. Wax baths and hydrotherapy may help. Synovectomy of diseased joint may improve function. Ruptured tendons in hand require repair. Arthrodesis of smaller joints may be helpful. Secondary osteoarthritis common.

Osteoarthritis

Degenerative wear-and-tear disease affects any joint but always one that has been under stress. Lower limbs affected more than upper.

Primary osteoarthritis occurs middle age onwards. Being overweight is only predisposing cause.

Secondary osteoarthritis may follow interference with blood supply to joints, e.g. Perthes' disease, fractures, traumatic dislocations, or interference with joint surfaces – congenital dislocation of the hip, infective arthritis, tuberculosis, slipped upper femoral epiphysis, rheumatoid arthritis, fractures and surgery. Articular cartilage, normally $\frac{1}{8}$ inch thick, frays and becomes fibrillated and may disappear altogether exposing bone. Synovial membrane becomes thicker and more vascular and protrudes into joint folds. Capsule thickens and contracts giving diminished movement. Bone hardens and increases in density and where exposed eburnates forming shiny surface. Osteophytes appear at periphery of bone. Cysts may form in bone: if numerous cause collapse of bone (Fig. 1.1).

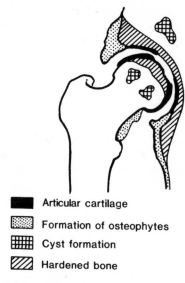

◼ Articular cartilage

▨ Formation of osteophytes

▦ Cyst formation

▨ Hardened bone

Fig. 1.1 Osteoarthritic changes in a hip joint. Note loss of joint space and wearing of articular cartilage.

Onset is gradual. Patient complains of pain and joint giving way. Pain not localised and often referred, e.g. hip pain felt in back and knee. Swelling not marked but may occur where there is little skin cover e.g. Heberden's nodes on finger joints.

X-ray shows loss of joint space, sclerosis of bone, lipping of bone edges with osteophyte formation and maybe formation of cysts.

Treatment. No known means of arresting degenerative process. General methods – Analgesics and anti-inflammatory drugs for pain. Weight reduction to reduce stress on joint. Local methods – Preservation of movements with physiotherapy and manipulations. Supply of crutches, sticks, corsets, collars, etc., as required. Hydrocortisone injections into joint help ease pain but increase rate of degeneration.

Operative methods – Four main types of operation used: osteotomy, arthrodesis, arthroplasty and excision arthroplasty. (Descriptions – see below.)

Osteotomy

Surgical cutting of bone. Used to correct angulation, bowing or rotation in a long bone, to help correct discrepancies in limb length. In case of arthritic joint, displacement osteotomy alters weight-bearing angle through joint and provides new weight-bearing surface (Fig. 1.2).

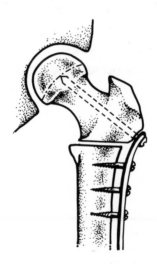

Fig. 1.2 Intertrochanteric displacement osteotomy with pin and plate fixation

Fractured bone ends following an osteotomy are usually held with internal fixation but splintage may be adequate. Weight is kept off joint until union is sound.

Arthrodesis

Fusion of joint abolishes pain at expense of movement. Greater strain placed on surrounding joints. Thought must be given to position of joint arthrodesis to allow optimum function. Operation particularly useful following tuberculosis or infective arthritis of joint when joint ends are severely damaged. Also useful for small joints in rheumatoid arthritis and in osteoarthritis when pain disabling (Fig. 1.3).

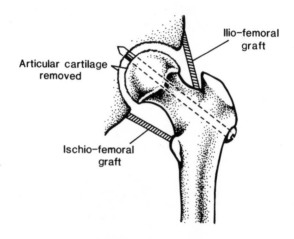

Fig. 1.3 Different ways in which a hip joint may be arthrodesed

Arthrodesis also used for correction of deformity, e.g. hammer toe and spinal curve after correction in structural scoliosis. When muscle power deficient as in poliomyelitis arthrodesis helps stabilise joint.

Arthroplasty

Surgical introduction of replacement joint. May be used for hip, knee, shoulder, elbow and finger joints. Great advance has been made in this field and more joints are becoming available. Prosthesis may be specially designed for patients with extensive malignant bone tumours.

Cup arthroplasty is used in hip to cover shaped head of femur. May be useful in younger person. When only femoral head damaged, e.g. following fracture, single component arthroplasty used – Thompson or Austin Moore prosthesis. For arthritic hips double replacements are used, often with metal portion in femur and plastic in acetabulum, e.g. Charnley, Stanmore, McKee-Farrar. Knee, shoulder and elbow joints are commonly all metal. Finger spacer joints are made of silastic material (Fig. 1.4).

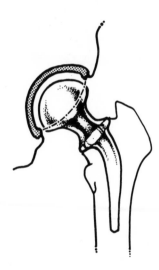

Fig. 1.4 Total hip arthroplasty with metal femoral component and plastic acetabular component

Following arthroplasty patient is mobilised quickly. Provides pain-free efficient joint.

Excision arthroplasty

One or both of articular ends of bone are removed creating a gap. Gap is filled with fibrous tissue or muscle stitched into position. Allows quite good range of movement but lacks stability. May be used on any joint on which an arthroplasty could be used except knee, e.g. Girdlestone's excision arthroplasty of hip, Keller's excision arthroplasty for hallux valgus (Fig. 1.5).

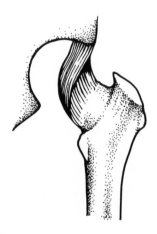

Fig. 1.5 Excision arthroplasty of hip (Girdlestone's operation)

Acute osteomyelitis

Occurs mainly in children but can affect adults. Infection, usually staphylococcus, reaches bone commonly through bloodstream from another septic focus or from external injury. If infection extends into joint it causes infective arthritis. Humerus, tibia and femur commonly affected. Rapid onset. General malaise with acute pain in affected bone. Often recent history of boil, injury or sore throat. X-rays do not show change at start of disease. Erythrocyte sedimentation rate and white cell count will be raised. Blood culture may be positive.

Treatment. Bed rest. Attempts to find causative organism by blood culture and culture of pus. Broad-spectrum antibiotics may be started until culture results available. Abscess may be drained to relieve tension. Limb splinted until disease quiescent. Long-term antibiotics.

Condition may become chronic with formation of sinus to skin. Sequestra (infected dead bone) may be removed to encourage healing.

TUMOURS

May be benign or malignant and affect bone cartilage, marrow or connective tissue.

Benign bone tumours

Osteoma, osteoid osteoma, osteoblastoma. Giant cell tumour – osteoclastoma – can become malignant and has tendency to recur.

Malignant bone tumour

Osteoasarcoma.

Benign cartilage tumours

Chondroma, osteochondroma, chondroblastoma.

Malignant cartilage tumours

Chondrosarcoma.

Malignant connective tissue tumour

Fibrosarcoma.

Marrow tumours

All malignant. Ewing's sarcoma, myeloma.

Treatment for benign tumours

Removal if causing pain, deformity or other problems or if there is any doubt of the histology.

Giant cell tumours appear most commonly in young adults, usually at the end of long bones. Regarded as potentially malignant.

Treatment. Careful curettage of tumour and packing with bone chips. Large tumours may be removed and prosthetic replacement inserted. Tendency of tumour to recur. If it becomes malignant, metastasises to lungs.

Treatment for malignant tumours

1. Osteosarcoma

Occurs most commonly in long bones of adolescents. Metastasises early, spreading to other bones and lungs.

Treatment. Bone scan to check for secondaries. Chemotherapy commenced. Amputation well above tumour or massive joint replacement in selected cases. Mortality rate very high. Frequent check-up's and scans essential.

2. Chondrosarcoma

Malignant tumour arising from cartilage. Less aggressive than osteosarcoma. Occurs most commonly in middle-aged people. Often seen in pelvis or shoulder girdle. Metastasises less rapidly than osteosarcoma.

Treatment. Excision of tumour whenever possible. Inaccessible sites treated with radiotherapy but tumours often resistant. Massive replacement may be possible. Forequarter or hindquarter amputation may be necessary for tumour in bony girdle.

3. Fibrosarcoma

Rare tumour arising from connective tissue. Found in long bones of young adults. Poor prognosis.

Treatment. Usually amputation combined with chemotherapy and/or radiotherapy.

4. Ewing's tumour

Dense tumour of long bone arising from marrow, found in children 5 to 16 years. New layers of bone form on top of tumour giving 'onion skin' appearance on X-ray.

Treatment. As for osteosarcoma.

5. Myelomatosis

Occurs in adults. Very common malignant condition of skeleton. Tumours probably arise from platelets and are spread to many bones via bloodstream. Patient generally ill and anaemic.

Treatment. Chemotherapy. Prognosis poor.

6. Secondary metastases of bone

Commonest malignant tumour of bone. Primary tumour may be carcinoma of breast, prostate, lung or thyroid. Pathological fractures may occur.

Treatment. Bone scans to diagnose site of primary and confirm other metastases. Analgesics, chemotherapy and maybe radiotherapy. Internal fixation of pathological fractures. Prognosis poor.

2

Trauma

FRACTURES

Fracture is interruption in continuity of bone. May be (a) complete, (b) incomplete (greenstick and crack). Caused by injury, stress, fatigue or underlying pathology.

Closed fractures – Bone is broken without damage to skin or outer tissues.

Open or compound fractures – Injury to skin at site of fracture giving direct access to bone for bacteria. Compound fractures may also be comminuted. Other tissues, nerves or blood vessels may be involved.

Signs and symptoms

1. Pain.
2. Loss of movement.
3. Swelling.
4. Deformity.
5. Crepitus.

First aid treatment. Primary splintage and transfer of patient to hospital as soon as possible.

Upper limbs – Support in sling or in front of coat, hold with uninjured arm or tie to side of body.

Lower limbs – Tie legs together padding bony prominences.

Pelvic, spinal or thoracic damage – Lift patient with extreme care, preferably on a blanket.

Jaw – Support with bandage or scarf. Ensure clean airway.
   Hospital treatment. General rules:
1. Maintain clear airway.
2. Treat for shock.
3. Arrest bleeding.
4. Cover compound fracture wounds.
5. Alleviate pain.
   Local treatment. Fractured limb is splinted using padded wooden or pneumatic splints. Always immobilise joint above and below fracture. X-rays taken as soon as possible.

Fractured clavicle

Common injury in all age groups.
   Treatment. Collar and cuff sling usually sufficient to control fracture. Normally heals readily. If displacement gross, internal fixation necessary. Bone ends held with wire until union complete and then removed. Exercises of shoulder very important.

Fractured scapula

Uncommon injury.
   Treatment. Injured arm supported in sling until pain lessens. Shoulder and arm exercises essential.

Fractures of the humerus

Fractured neck of humerus

Common fracture in the elderly. Fracture is often impacted.
   Treatment. Heals by gravity. Arm supported in collar and cuff sling. Finger, wrist and elbow exercises started immediately. Shoulder exercised as soon as possible.

Fractured shaft of humerus

Common to all ages.

Treatment. Manipulation rarely necessary. Fracture supported with 'U' slab plaster extending from shoulder to below elbow and bandaged into position. Arm supported in collar and cuff sling.

Complication. Radial nerve injury causing drop wrist.

Supracondylar fracture of humerus

Very common fracture in children.

Treatment. Undisplaced fracture immobilised in above elbow plaster. Radial pulse must be accessible. Child observed for at least 24 hours. Report immediately any pain, impairment of movement or change in circulation in fingers.

Complication. See Chapter 4. Extreme risk of damage to brachial artery resulting in Volkmann's ischaemic contracture. Median nerve may also be damaged.

Fractures of the forearm

Fractured olecranon

Common in adults.

Treatment. Undisplaced fractures immobilised in plaster. Displaced fractures may require screw fixation and splintage.

Fractured ulna with dislocation of radial head (Monteggia fracture)

Treatment. Reduction by open or closed methods. Splintage with above elbow plaster.

Fractured shaft of radius and/or ulna

Common to all ages. Children often sustain greenstick fractures.

Treatment. Closed reduction under anaesthetic with plaster splintage above elbow. Internal metal fixation may be necessary.

Fractured lower end of radius (Colles' fracture)

Common fracture, particularly in elderly. Caused by fall on outstretched hand. Fracture of distal end of radius and ulnar styloid. Radial fracture pulled backwards causing 'dinnerfork' deformity (Fig. 2.1). (Smith's fracture has opposite deformity. Radial fracture moves forwards towards palm.)

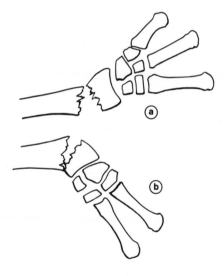

Fig. 2.1 Bony deformity in (a) Colles' fracture, (b) Smith's fracture

Treatment. Closed reduction under anaesthetic usual. Padded below-elbow plaster or backslab applied. Sling may be worn for 48 hours. Exercise of all other joints essential. Careful plaster instructions given to patient on discharge.

Complication. Redisplacement common. Progress watched weekly by X-rays.

Fractured scaphoid

Commonest carpal bone to be injured. Fracture often overlooked.

Treatment. Immobilisation in scaphoid plaster extending from first metacarpophalangeal joint to elbow. Other metacarpal joints left free.

Complication. Delayed union. Bone grafting may be necessary.

Fractured metacarpals

Common fractures following falls or fights. Fracture of first metacarpal involves carpometacarpal joint (Bennett's fracture).

Treatment. Often difficult to retain adequate reduction and internal fixation may be necessary. Undisplaced fractures of metacarpals require little or no splintage but need exercise. Displaced fractures may require reduction and splintage with malleable aluminium strip.

Fractured phalanges

Fingers stiffen quickly and must never be splinted for more than three weeks.

Treatment. Good immobilisation obtained by strapping fractured digit to next, allowing joint movements. Immobilise displaced fracture with malleable aluminium strip.

Crush fracture of distal phalanx

Disregard fracture and treat skin and soft tissue injury. Evacuate haematoma from under nail.

Fractured pelvis

Fractures not affecting continuity of pelvic ring

Fractures of pubic rami, ilium and into acetabulum.

Treatment. Rest in bed with exercise to lower limbs.

Complication. Rare with minor fractures but bladder damage must always be considered (Fig. 2.2).

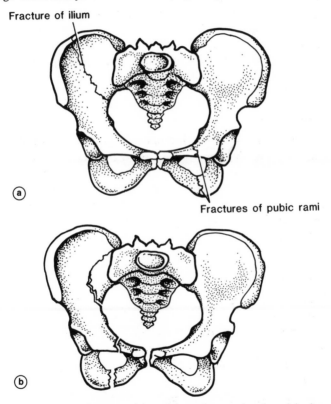

Fig. 2.2 (a) Stable fractures of the pelvis not interrupting the pelvic ring. (b) Double fracture of pubic rami and ilium causing interruption to pelvic ring

Fractures disrupting pelvic ring

Can be very serious.

Treatment. Rest with traction to legs if necessary. If pelvic bones have separated wide slings are used to support pelvis.

Complication. Bladder and urethra easily damaged. Urgent repair necessary.

Fractures of the femur

Fractured neck of femur

Common fracture in elderly. Complicated by minimal blood supply to femoral head. Fracture may be impacted (Fig. 2.3).

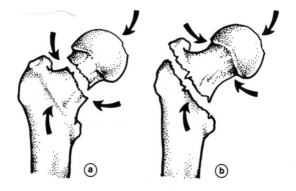

Fig. 2.3 (a) Fracture of neck of femur; (b) Intertrochanteric fracture of femur. Arrows indicate directions of blood supply

Treatment. Early surgery required. Patient made comfortable while waiting with Hamilton Russell traction. Fracture may be pinned but because of avascular necrosis, more commonly a prosthesis is inserted, e.g. Thompson or Austin Moore. Impacted fracture in younger person may be treated with Moore or Newman pins (Fig. 2.4).

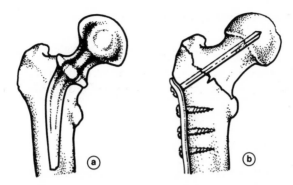

Fig. 2.4 Surgical treatment for fractured neck of femur. (a) Austin Moore prosthesis for fracture of neck of femur. (b) Pin and plate fixation for intertrochanteric fracture

Trochanteric fracture of femur

Common fracture in elderly. Blood supply to this area is better.

Treatment. Fracture is commonly pinned and plated. Encourage very early mobilisation to prevent chest and urinary infections and stiffness of other joints in elderly.

Fractured shaft of femur

Common fracture at all ages.

Treatment. May be conservative or surgical.

Conservative – Combination of upper tibial skeletal traction used with either Thomas' splint or Hamilton Russell traction. Fractures take at least three months to unite. Cast bracing may be used which helps promote early mobility and stimulates callus formation. Caliper protection may be necessary for severe fractures until bone soundly healed.

Surgical – Intramedullary nail, e.g. Kuntscher, hammered down shaft of femur. Method of choice if fracture is pathological in origin or if early mobilisation is required as in elderly.

Small children – both legs immobilised on gallows or similar traction.

Fracture heals in four to six weeks. Knees must be kept slightly flexed to prevent hyperextension of knee and subsequent arterial damage.

Supracondylar fracture of femur

Treatment. Conservative if fracture undisplaced. Leg rested in Thomas' splint. Good alignment of knee important. Displaced fractures require open reduction and insertion of blade plate and screws to hold fragments.

Fractured femoral condyles

Rare injury.

Treatment. Traction and conservative treatment often adequate but insertion of screw may be required to prevent knee damage.

Fractured patella

Treatment. Undisplaced fractures held in plaster cylinder. Displaced fractures require surgery. In younger patients fragments bolted together. Patella excised in older patients.

Fractures of the tibia and fibula

Fractured tibial condyles

Difficult to manage, often complicated by haemarthrosis. Late osteoarthritis likely because of damage to articular surface.

Treatment. Fracture usually treated by rest and splintage. Manipulation under anaesthetic may be needed.

Fractured shaft of tibia and fibula

Due to nearness of tibia to skin, fractures are often compound. Important to obtain good end to end alignment of tibia to prevent shortening or deformity. Majority of patients require admission because of swelling. Elevation and observation of toes essential.

Treatment. Undisplaced fracture held in long leg plaster. Limb must be non-weight bearing for minimum of three weeks. Displaced fracture may need skeletal traction, e.g. Steinmann pin through calcaneum with leg supported on a Braun's frame (Fig. 2.6). Internal fixation may be used, either intramedullary nail or screws. Compound fractures require immediate attention. May be difficult to suture wounds due to lack of viable skin. Skin grafts may be necessary at later stage. Severly comminuted fractures may be held in place with external fixation apparatus, e.g. Hoffman's frame.

Fractured ankle

Common fractures. May displace mortise joint with or without dislocation (Pott's fracture) (Fig. 2.5).

Treatment. Fractures without displacement of mortise joint usually managed in below-knee plaster. Displaced fractures require manipulation to obtain reduction and are then held

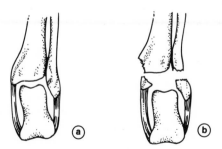

Fig. 2.5 (a) Mortise joint construction at ankle. (b) Fracture-dislocation of ankle joint

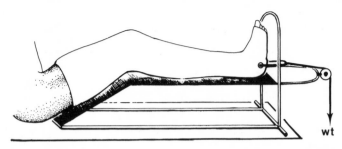

Fig. 2.6 Use of skeletal traction through calcaneum, combined with high elevation on a Braun's frame, for fractured shaft of tibia

in below-knee plaster. Internal fixation screws may be necessary to hold displaced malleolus. High elevation required, swelling may be gross, sometimes necessitating splitting or change of plaster.

Fractures of the foot

Fractured talus

Uncommon but can be difficult to treat.

Treatment. Below-knee plaster to hold fracture after reduction.

Complication. Malunion and avascular necrosis common.

Fractured calcaneus

Commonly caused by fall on to heel.

Treatment. Simple fracture requires rest in below-knee plaster. Crush fracture treated with rest and elevation. Gravitational oedema common if foot not kept highly elevated. Important to exercise all other joints.

Fractured metatarsals

Treatment. Fractures heal readily but usually held in below-knee plaster for pain relief.

Stress fracture of metatarsal (March fracture)

Commonly occurs in shaft of second or third metatarsal.
Treatment. Symptomatic.

Fractured phalanges

Require no treatment except elevation to alleviate pain and prevent knocks.

Fracture of spinal column

Fractures involving spinal column can be extremely serious, especially if complicated by damage to spinal cord with resulting paraplegia or quadriplegia. Any damage to neck or back regarded as serious until proved otherwise. All patients should be lifted by three persons with a fourth supporting the head.

Fractured transverse process or crush fracture of body of vertebra

Treatment. These give localised back pain. Patient nursed freely in bed. Help with turning may be necessary for first few days.

Fracture dislocation of cervical spine

Very serious. Usually results in quadraplegia.
Treatment. Patient nursed flat and skeletal cervical traction applied. Weights increased until X-ray shows reduction of dislocation and then gradually reduced. Traction maintained for six weeks. Patient then up in brace and commences physio- and occupational therapy. Persistent instability of dislocation may require cervical fusion.

Fractured thoracic or lumbar spine with cord involvement

Treatment. Traction unnecessary. Patient nursed flat in bed for six weeks. Then up in brace and commences rehabilitation. Unstable spine may be fused and supported with Harrington rod.

Nursing care of paraplegic and quadraplegic patients

Damage to the spinal cord produces loss of skin sensation. Essential to turn patients two to three hourly to prevent skin ischaemia and resultant pressure sores. Important to prevent limb deformities by good positioning, support and passive physiotherapy. Bladder emptying controlled by indwelling catheter until general condition of patient is stable. Different methods of treatment for bladder control. Method of choice may be sterile intermittent catheterisation. Patient catheterised five times daily. Paraplegic patients taught to do this themselves; member of family may be taught procedure for quadraplegic. Fluids very important while patient has indwelling catheter but may be limited to 1500 ml daily for intermittent catheterisation patients. Bowel control taught by administration of suppositories every other day. Manual evacuation may be required initially to stimulate bowel to empty. Rehabilitation commenced after six weeks when patient allowed up in brace. Tilting bed may be used to re-educate patient to an erect position. Physio- and occupational therapy essential for patient to learn and adapt to new way of life. Return to community made as soon as possible. Adaptations made to homes to accommodate wheelchair. Patients often very depressed on realisation of their life ahead. A great deal of help and encouragement is required from the whole team of people who work with spinal injury patients, not only while they are in hospital but also when the patient is home and attempting to cope in the community.

Fractures in thoracic cage

Pain made worse by respiratory movements.

Treatment. No special treatment. Severe pain may be relieved by infiltration with local anaesthetic. Maintenance of airway and treatment of complications far more important than the fractures.

Complications. Pneumothorax, haemothorax, pneumonia and surgical emphysema.

Complications of fractures

1. Delayed or malunion.
2. Deformity or shortening with resulting pain.
3. Infection.
4. Injury to blood vessels or nerves.
5. Avascular necrosis.
6. Osteoarthritis.
7. Fat embolus.

DISLOCATIONS AND SUBLUXATIONS

Dislocation occurs when the joint surfaces are moved in such a way that joint apposition is lost.

Subluxation occurs when the joint surface apposition is partially lost.

Signs and symptoms

1. Pain.
2. Swelling.
3. Loss of movement.

Clinical feature of deformity usually confirms diagnosis. Strain of a joint is damage to the ligaments.

Acromioclavicular joint

May be dislocated, subluxed or strained.

Treatment. Subluxations and strains treated with a sling and early active exercises. Dislocation more difficult to hold and often requires internal fixation for short period until ligaments have healed.

Shoulder

Dislocation common in adults but not in children. Usually caused by fall on outstretched hand. May be anterior or posterior dislocation but most commonly anterior.

Treatment. Reduction usually requires anaesthetic. Sling used to support arm and early active exercises necessary.

Complication. Damage to axillary nerve producing paralysis of deltoid muscle.

Elbow

Dislocation fairly common in all age groups.

Treatment. Reduction requires anaesthetic followed by above-elbow plaster with elbow held at 90°.

Complication. Rare. Joint stiffness common.

Subluxation head of radius (pulled elbow)

Very common injury to children. Caused by pulling hard on hand.

Treatment. Easily reduced without anaesthetic.

Dislocations of carpal bones

Commonest is dislocation of lunate.

Treatment. Reduction under anaesthetic necessary and plaster immobilisation.

Dislocation of finger joints

Treatment. Usually reduced without anaesthetic. No immobilisation.

Dislocation of hip

Common injury following road traffic accident. Often combined with femoral or acetabular fractures.

Treatment. Reduction as soon as possible under anaesthetic. Traction such as Hamilton Russell maintains hip position whilst healing.

Complication. Injury to sciatic nerve. Osteoarthritis.

Dislocation of knee

Rare injury as knee is well supported by strong ligaments.

Treatment. Reduction under anaesthetic. Immobilisation in long leg plaster.

Complication. Damage to popliteal artery.

Dislocation of patella

Injury can be isolated incident or recurrent.

Treatment. Reduced easily. Robert Jones' bandage for support. Effusion of knee usually occurs. Recurrent dislocation more common in girls. If disabling, surgery performed: transposition of patellar tendon. See Chapter 6.

Knee ligaments

Tears of medial, lateral or cruciate may occur.

Treatment. Usually conservative with short term immobilisation in plaster followed by active exercises.

Menisci of knee (semilunar cartilages)

Commonly torn especially in young men and athletes. Patient

experiences pain and inability to straighten knee after twisting injury.

Treatment. Initially knee straightened, with anaesthetic if necessary. Supported in Robert Jones' bandage. Recurrent episodes necessitate meniscectomy. See Chapter 6.

Ankle

Dislocation without fracture is rare.

Treatment. As fracture: reduction and splintage.

Ruptured lateral ligaments of ankle

Strain-view X-rays taken to differentiate from less severe injury.

Treatment. Long-term plaster conservative treatment required to prevent recurrent subluxation of ankle.

Strained lateral ligaments of ankle

Treatment. Strapping or crepe support required for two weeks minimum.

Ruptured Achilles tendon

May occur whilst running or jumping. Rupture always complete.

Treatment. Suturing of tendon required for good result. Plaster applied with foot in plantar flexion for three weeks, then new plaster with foot at 90°.

3

Splintage and traction

PLASTER SPLINTAGE

Plaster of Paris is made from gypsum and supplied as prepared bandages of different widths, as plaster slabs or as a powder which may be mixed to form a cream.

Correctly applied plaster of Paris gives very good splintage for fractures. Also used to correct deformities and give rest and support to injured or diseased parts of the skeleton.

Application of plaster

Padded plasters should be applied for all new fractures and following surgery. Stockingette may be used over the skin. Padding applied over joints and bony prominences with wool, e.g. Orthoban. Larger areas, e.g. pelvic crests, protected with felt.

Plaster application is a skilled procedure and needs a lot of practice to be successful. Plaster bandage or slab soaked in warm water and excess water squeezed out before applying. (N.B. Always hold end of bandage between thumb and forefinger prior to soaking.) Wet plaster is moulded to body during application to ensure one solid cast and not separate layers. Edges of completed plaster either covered with stockingette and held in place or trimmed to prevent roughness and to allow joint movement above and below the plaster.

Drying of plaster

Wet plaster is very vulnerable and must be handled with great care. Dry on blanket on top of plastic-covered pillow. Turn regularly using palms of hands to prevent finger dents. Limbs in plaster should be elevated. Do not use external heat to dry plaster.

Observations

Observe patient generally and, in case of plaster on limb, watch extremities. Pain, change of colour or loss of movement in digits must be reported immediately. Higher elevation may help situation and doctor may advise 'splitting' of plaster to relieve tension.

Instructions for outpatients

Every plaster applied on casualty or outpatient should be checked next day. Written instructions must be given advising immediate return to hospital if plaster is tight, digits are blue or cold, or there is severe pain. Advice also given about drying plaster, not to wet it or push objects down it and to keep other joints fully active.

Plaster sores

All reports of intense itching, burning or pain must be investigated. Plaster should be windowed and area of skin inspected. If skin is broken and requires dressing, plaster window held in place with strapping. If window is left off, skin will swell through window and cause further pressure.

If sores not detected at early stage they may be noticed by the smell, staining of plaster and patient being generally unwell. A small child may be fretful and feverish.

Removal of plaster

When possible it is removed with plaster shears, the lower blade of the shears being kept between the plaster and padding. Plaster saw may be necessary for thick plaster jackets or hip spicas.

Plaster beds

Made using sheets of muslin and plaster cream. Posterior half of shell moulded over back of patient from neck to ankles. When dry it is mounted on frame and pillow support made. Hooks are attached to frame for swinging purposes. Anterior shell made from base of neck to ankles and mounted in same way. To turn patient, swinging cords are removed, anterior shell is strapped into place and patient turned completely over. Posterior half then removed. Reverse procedure to turn patient back. It is kind to warm the spare half of plaster before turning.

Cast bracing (Fig. 3.1)

A modern form of hinged cast used particularly following fractures of femoral shaft. Carefully applied with hinges at the knee. Earlier mobilisation possible. Added weight through fracture site increases rate of callus formation. Early mobilisation is good psychological boost. Also allows free exercise of hip and knee.

Splintage other than plaster of Paris

New techniques and materials are being introduced all the time as means of splintage and support. Light synthetic materials, e.g. Hexelite, Baycast or Scotchcast, all have different properties for drying, early weight bearing and lightness of

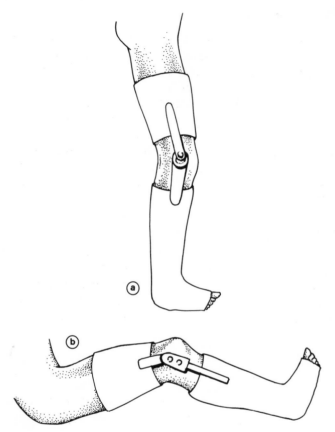

Fig. 3.1 (a) Cast-brace for fractured shaft of femur. (b) Flexion that can be obtained at knee joint

cast. Material selected to suit cast required. Some of these materials can only be removed with a plaster saw.

Plastazote and Ortholene are excellent materials for making collars and splints. They are heated and moulded to the patient or a cast of the patient. Appliances may be held in place with press-studs or Velcro straps.

TRACTION

Traction may be necessary to correct alignment of bones following fracture or dislocation, to correct congenital abnormalities prior to surgery or to provide relief for back pain. It may be skin or skeletal traction.

Skin traction – Applied outside limb using elastoplast or Ventfoam extensions and bandaged into place. Requires regular checking and rebandaging.

Skeletal traction – Steinmann or Denham pin inserted through bone and traction applied. Used when a lot of pull is required, e.g. when strong muscles pull fracture out of line.

Hamilton Russell traction (Fig. 3.2)

May be used with skin or skeletal traction. Skeletal used for fractures of shaft of femur, fractures or dislocations of the hip joint or whenever a strong pull on the femur or hip is required. Steinmann pin usually sited through tibial condyles. Skin traction, Elastoplast or Ventfoam used when lesser pull

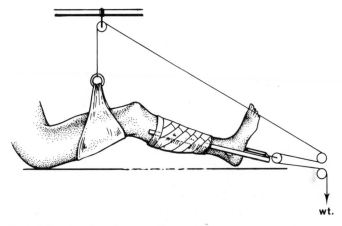

wt.

Fig. 3.2 Hamilton Russell using skin extensions

required, e.g. to mobilise hip and knee after period in plaster or for patients with fractured neck of femur awaiting surgery.

Thomas' splint

May be used with skin or skeletal traction. With skeletal traction may be used for fractures of femur. Knee injuries or condylar fractures can be supported in splint when skin extensions may be applied. Splint may be used purely to rest leg, e.g. osteomyelitis. Used to protect and rest leg after insertion of massive replacement prostheses for tumour surgery.

Slings and spring traction (Fig. 3.3)

A simple and effective traction to rest and mobilise leg at the same time. Sling supports under thigh and calf attached to overhead bar by long springs. Allows movement at all joints. Particularly useful following hip surgery or leg lengthening. Springs of different strength may be used to increase muscle power.

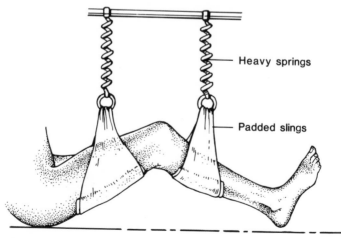

— Heavy springs

— Padded slings

Fig. 3.3 Slings and springs traction

Pelvic traction

Used for low back pain. Well-fitting corset attached by straps to spreader bar beyond feet. Central cord passes from spreader over swan-neck pulley to weights.

Skeletal head traction

Used for cervical lesions, to reduce fracture dislocations of cervical spine and in combination with other forms of traction as method of correction in scoliosis. Half halo with four pins may be used or skull calipers, e.g. Crutchfield tongs.

Halter traction

Used for neck lesions. Leather or disposable halter attached to single metal bar above head. Cord attached from bar over swan-neck pulley to weights. May be used in lying or sitting position.

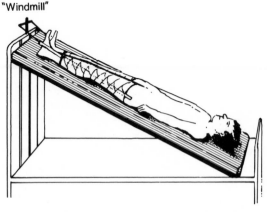

"Windmill"

Fig. 3.4 Pugh's traction

Pugh's traction (Fig. 3.4)

Used to aid correction of some congenital deformities, e.g. congenital dislocation of hip and some scoliosis prior to surgery. Fracture board is tied firmly to head of bed. Patient is placed with head to foot end of bed. Either lower tibial skeletal pins or Elastoplast skin extensions are used to exert traction on legs. No weights are used. Gravity aids correction of pelvic tilt for scoliosis and helps pull a dislocated hip nearer the acetabulum. Traction sickness may be a problem initially. Problem alleviated by raising foot of bed (patient's head) and lowering it gradually over twenty-four hours.

Stryker frames

Specially adapted turning bed used when traction must be maintained whilst patient is turned. Used especially for correction of severe scoliosis prior to surgery. Also used for spinal injuries or following other spinal surgery. Traction may be applied to head, feet or both. Head usually held with half-halo or skull calipers. Leg traction obtained using lower tibial pins or skin extensions.

Cotrel traction

Specially designed traction used to stretch and mobilise the spine prior to fusion in scoliosis. Used intermittently through the day. When patient stretches legs downwards, the halter and weights stretch the head away from the body thus stretching the spine. X-ray may be taken in stretched position to show mobility of the spine. Possible to record weight exerted on spine which assists surgeon at time of fusion (Figs 3.5 and 3.6).

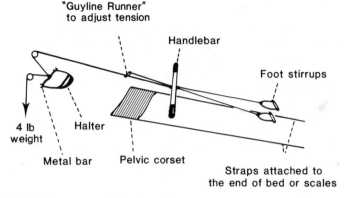

Fig. 3.5 Components of Cotrel traction

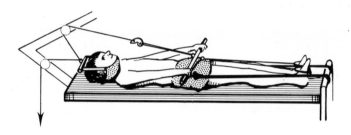

Fig. 3.6 Cotrel traction in use

GENERAL CARE OF PATIENTS WEARING CALIPERS, APPLIANCES OR BRACES

Any skin marking or rubbing must be reported and if possible area to be seen by orthotist so that accurate adjustment can be made. Modern appliances are as streamlined and cosmetic as possible but patients still need help, encouragement and education to wear them correctly and thus gain maximum benefit.

4

Conditions affecting the neck and upper limbs

THE NECK AND CERVICAL SPINE

Cervical spine is most mobile part of vertebral column. Neck diseases often affect nerve roots of brachial plexus and cause symptoms in upper limbs.

Torticollis

Infantile torticollis – see Chapter 7.

Tuberculosis of cervical spine

Uncommon condition.

Treatment (see Chapter 1). Fusion may be necessary in quiescent stage.

Infective arthritis of cervical spine

Rare condition.

Treatment (see Chapter 1). Spontaneous fusion of vertebrae may occur.

Osteoarthritis of cervical spine

Common site for degenerative changes, may be initiated by injury. Pain in back of neck and trapezius muscle; crepitus (grating) on movement. Referred pain or weakness in upper limbs. In very severe cases osteophytes may form and press on spinal cord causing paralysis.

Treatment (see Chapter 1). Analgesics, manipulation under anaesthetic and physiotherapy, rest and support in collar. Very severe cases may require fusion of affected vertebrae.

Prolapsed cervical disc

Uncommon site for prolapse but may occur as acute episode or come on gradually. Usually follows injury. Myelography confirms diagnosis.

Treatment. Conservative – rest, collar and analgesics. Traction may help and exercises once pain has subsided. A few patients require surgical decompression of the cord.

Extra cervical rib

Congenital anomaly; may cause neurological or vascular symptoms in upper limbs.

Treatment. Removal of rib if symptoms are severe.

Tumours of cervical spine

Benign tumours are rare. Malignant tumours may involve spinal cord, meninges, nerves or bone. Tumours in apex of lung may spread into neck.

Treatment. Removal if possible, radiotherapy and cytotoxic drugs. Stability of cervical spine maintained with collar for as long as possible.

THE SHOULDER REGION

The shoulder is made up of glenohumeral, acromioclavicular and sternoclavicular joints.

Tuberculosis of shoulder

Rare site of infection.

Treatment (see Chapter 1). Active exercises as soon as possible. Arthrodesis may be performed if joint destroyed.

Infective arthritis of shoulder

Uncommon condition.

Treatment (see Chapter 1). Active exercises as soon as joint has settled.

Rheumatoid arthritis of shoulder

Not a commonly affected joint.

Treatment (see Chapter 1). Very important to exercise and maintain movement of joint.

Osteoarthritis of shoulder

Rare site for osteoarthritis but may occur after injury or disease.

Treatment (see Chapter 1). Usually conservative. Very severe cases may require arthrodesis or total replacement.

Recurrent dislocation of shoulder

Initial traumatic dislocation may weaken joint and lead to recurrent anterior dislocation.

Treatment. Surgery is required; there are two common operations.

Bankart's operation – capsule is re-attached to front of joint.

Putti–Platt operation – subscapularis tendon is shortened to limit lateral rotation.

Frozen shoulder

Adhesive capsulitis. Painful condition. Unknown cause. Pain and limitation of all movements.

Treatment. Conservative. Rest in acute stages. Relief of pain with analgesics and maybe anti-inflammatory drugs. Passive exercises in acute stages and then active physiotherapy as soon as pain allows. Injection of hydrocortisone with local anaesthetic into the joint may increase rate of pain relief. Manipulation under anaesthetic helpful in some cases. Full recovery normally takes many months.

Painful arc syndrome

Pain experienced when shoulder abducted between 60° and 120°. May be due to damage or tendonitis of rotator cuff, or calcification in supraspinatus tendon.

Treatment. Inflamed tendons relieved with injection of hydrocortisone and local anaesthetic. Severe tears of rotator cuff require repair. Calcification often resolves with steroid injection but some require removal of deposit.

THE UPPER ARM

Upper arm more prone to injury than disease.

Acute osteomyelitis of humerus

Less common in upper limb than lower but occurs mainly in children.

Treatment (see Chapter 1). Drainage of abscess if necessary.

Tumours of upper arm

Benign giant cell tumour (osteoclastoma) may develop, usually at upper end. Removal advised but tumour may reform. Tendency to become malignant. Radical excision or total prosthetic replacement may be necessary. Malignant tumours rare in upper limb. Secondary metastatic tumours often appear in humerus. Pathological fractures are common.

THE ELBOW

Elbow in full extension is normally slightly valgus – 10° in men, 15° in women, to form carrying angle. Previous injury, surgery or infection may alter angle.

Cubitus valgus

Degree of valgus increased. Ulnar nerve may be affected in severe cases.

Treatment. If angulation severe or ulnar nerve affected, osteotomy of lower end of humerus.

Cubitus varus

Carrying angle decreased but no nerve involvement.

Treatment. Osteotomy of lower end of humerus if deformity disfiguring.

Tuberculosis of elbow

Not a common site for tuberculosis.

Treatment (see Chapter 1). Active exercises as soon as disease has subsided. If joint destroyed, arthrodesis or arthroplasty may be necessary.

Infective arthritis of elbow

Elbow may be infected due to external wound, blood-borne infection or from site of osteomyelitis nearby.

Treatment (see Chapter 1). Active exercise as soon as possible.

Rheumatoid arthritis of elbow

Common site of disease.

Treatment (see Chapter 1). Surgery may be needed for severe joint damage. Arthrodesis in position of optimum function or arthroplasty performed.

Osteoarthritis of elbow

May occur following injury, disease or surgery. Osteophytes may become detached forming loose bodies which can cause elbow to lock.

Treatment (see Chapter 1). Conservative treatment where possible. Loose bodies may be removed with relief. Arthrodesis or arthroplasty performed if joint damage very severe.

Osteochondritis dissecans of elbow

Common site of disease. There is necrosis of part of the articular cartilage and bone. Bone fragments may separate and form loose bodies.

Treatment. The loose bodies are removed when they have separated.

'Tennis elbow'

Pain and acute tenderness laterally outside elbow joint.

Treatment. Injection of hydrocortisone and local anaesthetic into point of greatest tenderness. Pain often increases before improvement. Physiotherapy helps restore full movement.

Ulnar neuritis

Ulnar nerve may be submitted to friction at elbow joint, e.g. cubitus valgus or osteoarthritis. Numbness or tingling experienced in fingers supplied by ulnar nerve.

Treatment. Surgical transposition of ulnar nerve to front of joint.

THE WRIST AND HANDS

Many symptoms in hands are caused by neck disorders.

Infective arthritis of wrist

Uncommon condition.

Treatment (see Chapter 1). Active movement as soon as infection settles.

Infective arthritis of fingers

Any finger joint may be involved, usually following external injury.

Treatment. As for wrist.

Rheumatoid arthritis of wrist and hands

Rheumatoid arthritis commonly affects wrists and hands and may cause serious loss of function and deformity. Joints are swollen, painful and movement restricted. Articular cartilage and bone may be eroded causing fingers to deviate towards ulna. Tendons may rupture.

Treatment (see Chapter 1). In acute phases wrist only may be splinted at night. Physiotherapy and occupational therapy help to preserve finger movement. Surgically, synovectomy may slow down rate of progression of disease. Ruptured tendons may be repaired or replaced. Arthroplasty to insert metal or Silastic finger joints. Arthrodesis of wrist or individual finger joints can stabilise joint and ease pain.

Osteoarthritis of wrist

This is most common after injury to wrist, e.g. fractured scaphoid or secondary to rheumatoid arthritis.

Treatment. Preferably conservative but if pain very severe arthrodesis of wrist in position of optimum function.

Osteoarthritis of fingers

Affects distal interphalangeal joints and carpometacarpal joint of thumb. Swellings known as Heberden's nodes.

Treatment. Usually conservative. Analgesics for pain. If finger of thumb deformity very severe, joint may be fused in position of function.

Osteochondritis of lunate (Kienböck's disease)

Cause unknown; may be deficiency in blood supply or repeated injury. Causes pain, reduction in grip and limitation of movement. Very likely to develop osteoarthritis at a later date.

Treatment. Plaster splintage often unsatisfactory.

Surgery – excision of lunate is successful if prior to development of osteoarthritis.

Tenosynovitis of wrist

Tendons at back of forearm inflamed, usually due to repeated use and excessive friction of tendons. Local swelling and pain on movement. Crepitus (grating) may be felt over swelling.

Treatment. Rest and splintage for up to 3 months.

Tumours of hand

Benign chondroma tumours may occur in metacarpals or phalanges.

Treatment. Surgically removed if any doubt of diagnosis.

Volkmann's ischaemic contracture

Flexion deformity of wrist and fingers caused by ischaemia of flexor muscles due to injury of brachial artery (see Chapter 2). Most common in children. If arterial obstruction not observed, fingers are white and cold and radial pulse absent. Finger movement is painful, contracture develops over weeks.

Treatment. At time of injury, hand and pulse must be observed. If arterial obstruction suspected all splints and bandages removed and warmth applied to improve circulation. If this fails, brachial artery must be explored without delay. Established contractures irreversible, can only be treated with reconstructive surgery – muscle and tendon transfers, wrist arthrodesis or nerve grafting.

Carpal tunnel syndrome

Compression of median nerve beneath flexor retinaculum. Common in middle-aged women. Tingling and numbness in fingers supplied by median nerve. Pain and tingling most commonly felt at night.

Treatment. Nerve is decompressed by division of flexor retinaculum.

Ganglion

Common harmless cystic swelling found on back of wrist.

Treatment. If disfiguring or interfering with nerve supply, may be removed.

Dupuytren's contracture (Fig. 4.1)

Flexion contracture of finger at metacarpophalangeal and interphalangeal joints. Due to shortening and thickening of palmar fascia. More common in men.

Treatment. Surgery if progression is rapid, excising thickened palmar fascia. Very severe contracture may be best treated by amputation of the finger concerned.

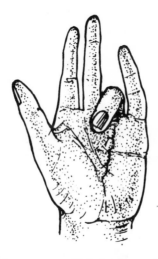

Fig. 4.1 Dupuytren's contracture of left ring finger with nodular thickening in the palm.

De Quervain's syndrome

Nodule in abductor pollicis longus and extensor pollicis longus due to thickening. Most common in middle-aged women. Pain on using hand and thumb.

Treatment. Rest and hydrocortisone injection gives slow recovery. Surgical incision of tendon sheaths gives quicker results.

Trigger finger

Thickening of tendon sheath preventing free movement of flexor tendons. Affects middle-aged women (finger) and babies (thumb). Finger locks in flexion and can only be straightened with difficulty. Infant's thumb locked in flexion.

Treatment. Surgical incision of flexor tendon sheaths.

Tendon injuries

Tendons may be cut or rupture.

Treatment. Usually necessary to repair tendons by direct suturing or replacing by grafting another tendon.

Mallet finger

Extensor tendon ruptures over distal interphalangeal joint, usually due to a blow on tip of finger.

Treatment. Finger splinted with distal interphalangeal joint in extension and proximal interphalangeal joint flexed. Surgery rarely required.

Sudek's atrophy

Condition which may follow any injury especially Colles' fracture, or surgery to upper arm. Cause unknown. Patient suffers severe pain, stiffness, oedema, shininess and vasodilation of hand and wrist. Later becomes cold and cyanotic. Bones become osteoporotic.

Treatment. Splintage, whilst very painful in position of function. Physiotherapy commenced as soon as pain allows. Very slow recovery. Injections of local anaesthetic or guanethidine blocks may help.

5

Conditions affecting thorax and spine

Tuberculosis of spine (Pott's disease)

Commonest site of bony tuberculosis infection. Invades vertebral body and often involves disc. Erosion of vertebra causes anterior collapse and angular kyphosis. Abscesses commonly form and may track down behind muscles, e.g. psoas abscess forms in iliac fossa. Untreated cases may develop severe kyphosis and there may be paraplegia.

Treatment (see Chapter 1). Spine must be rested in bed. Additional splintage by nursing patient in plaster bed if in severe pain. Abscesses require drainage. Paraplegia may be relieved by decompression of cord. Necrotic bone may be removed to aid healing process. Affected part of spine may be fused when disease quiescent, if necessary. Anti-tuberculous drug therapy continued for a minimum of a year, longer if there has been surgical intervention. Patient allowed up in spinal support once ESR has returned to normal. Rehabilitation is taken deliberately slowly.

Infection of thoracic or lumbar spine

Uncommon condition but if occurs usually due to Streptococcus or Staphylococcus. Similar symptoms to tuberculosis of spine. Abscesses may form. Identification of bacteria essential.

Treatment (see Chapter 1). Long-term rest for spine in bed or plaster bed and later in spinal jacket. Drainage of abscesses if necessary. Appropriate chemotherapy. Surgery unlikely but fusion may be required if vertebrae severely damaged.

Rheumatoid arthritis of spine

Vertebral joints often affected together with rest of skeleton.
Treatment – see Chapter 1.

Osteoarthritis of spine

Spine often affected, particularly in persons doing heavy work. Patients often complain of sudden acute attacks of lumbago pain which may last several weeks.

Treatment (see Chapter 1). Physiotherapy to strengthen spinal muscles. Lumbar pain may be helped by corset. Very severe cases helped by spinal fusion.

Osteochondritis of spine (Scheuermann's disease)

Adolescent kyphosis of unknown cause. Pain in thoracic region due to disturbance of growth in vertebrae. Kyphus of thoracic spine develops. There may be hyperlordosis of lumber spine. Subject to osteoarthritis in later life.

Treatment. Aim is to prevent increase in kyphus by holding it in either by a brace or a corrective plaster jacket. Established kyphus may require correction with Cotrel traction and fusion with bilateral Harrington compression rods.

Ankylosing spondylitis

Inflammatory condition of spine usually in men. Begins in sacroiliac joints and progresses upwards affecting all spinal joints. After inflammation joints ankylose, leaving bent stiff spine.

Treatment. Anti-inflammatory drugs, e.g. phenylbutazone. Physiotherapy to help maintain as much spinal movement as possible. Radiotherapy sometimes given but carries risk of leukaemia.

Benign tumours of spinal column

Rare condition. Aneurysmal bone cyst, a highly vascular cyst, may occur in vertebral body or spinous process in children.

Treatment. Removal of cyst if possible. Radiotherapy will usually cure it.

Malignant tumours of spinal column

Tumours may be primary, e.g. sarcoma or myeloma, but there are commonly metastases. May cause compression of spinal cord or destruction of vertebrae causing collapse of spine.

Treatment. Excision of primary tumour if possible. Analgesics, radiotherapy and cytotoxic drugs.

Prolapsed intervertebral disc

Very common condition. Discs between L4/L5 and L5/S1 vertebrae most commonly affected. Following injury, which may be slight, tear occurs in fibrous part of disc, annulus fibrosus (Fig. 5.1). The jelly-like nucleus pulposus may protrude through herniation and press on spinal cord causing generalised backache and acute sciatic pain. There may be sensory changes in calf and foot. Coughing and sneezing make pain worse. All back movements, particularly straight leg raising, are limited and painful.

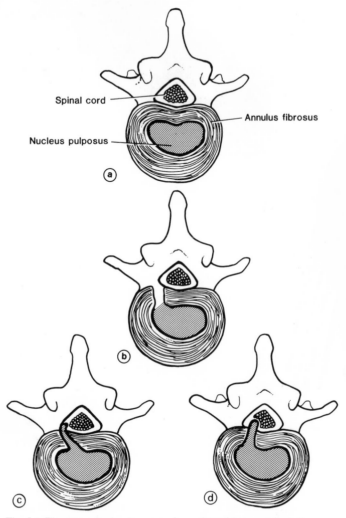

Fig. 5.1 The stages in development of a prolapsed intervertebral disc. (a) The normal disc. (b) The annulus fibrosus is torn. (c) Nucleus pulposus protrudes through the tear. (d) Nucleus protrudes further and presses on spinal cord and issuing nerve.

Treatment. Rest, flat in bed with board under mattress is often sufficient to allow nucleus pulposus to resume normal position. Pelvic traction may help process. Lumbar corset when up and about for support. Myelogram or radiculogram confirm diagnosis. If conservative treatment fails, offending nucleus pulposus and part of annulus fibrosus may be removed by surgery. Active physiotherapy necessary once wound healed.

Spondylolisthesis

Congenital defect of neural arch, usually of L5 with forward slip of vertebra on S1. Displacement may progress slowly during childhood and rapidly in adolescence. Neurological symptoms may occur.

Treatment. According to symptoms. Mild symptoms treated with corset. Severe neurological symptoms relieved by decompression of spinal nerve root and fusion of vertebrae.

Coccydynia

Pain in sacrococcygeal area usually following a fall. Pain especially on sitting can persist for many years.

Treatment. Exclusion of rectal disease. Reassurance to patient that pain will eventually resolve. Injection of hydrocortisone and local anaesthetic may help. If pain very severe coccyx may be removed.

Spina bifida

See Chapter 7.

Scoliosis

May be (a) postural or (b) structural.

stural: due to bad posture or tilted pelvis caused by
quality. No rotation of vertebral bodies. Apparent
curve corrects on flexion of spine.

(b) Structural: lateral curvature of the spine with rotation
of the vertebrae (Fig. 5.2). Classified according to cause if
known. 75% idiopathic, 25% cause known.

Origin may be:

Myogenic	– muscular disorders, e.g. muscular dystrophy.
Osteogenic	– congenital bony abnormalities, hemi-vertebrae, fused ribs, osteogenesis imperfecta.
Neurogenic	– diseases affecting the nervous system, e.g. poliomyelitis, neurofibromatosis, peroneal muscular atrophy, Friedreich's ataxia.
Thoracogenic	– due to previous thoracic surgery.
Idiopathic	– cause unknown. Largest group. Three age groups – infantile, juvenile and idiopathic.

Treatment

Many minor curves do not require treatment. AP X-ray of
spine taken and maximum angle of curve measured. Lateral
X-ray will show if kyphosis present. Spinal films repeated at
intervals, angles measured and progress of curve noted. Progression requires treatment.

Infantile scoliosis. Ninety per cent of curves resolve without
treatment. Progressive curves moulded and held in plaster lo-
caliser jacket or Milwaukee brace. Correction can be obtained
in the young child and the spine then grows straight. De-
teriorating curves require correction and surgery. Correction
obtained on Stryker frame using half halo and tibial pin traction. Anterior release may be performed followed two to three
weeks later by segmental posterior fusion.

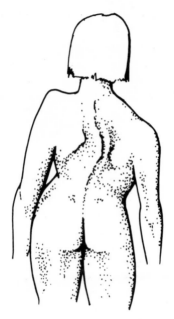

Fig. 5.2 Adolescent idiopathic scoliosis.

Juvenile and adolescent scoliosis. Minor curves watched in scoliosis clinic. Curves over 25° may be held in plaster, Milwaukee or ortholene brace until growth complete. Greater curves require correction and fusion. Mobile curves do not always require correction prior to surgery but Cotrel traction if used will increase mobility of spine and indicate the pressure which may be exerted through the spine. Stiff curves need skeletal traction on a Stryker frame. A halo chair may also be used. Mobile curves fused posteriorly using Harrington rod and bone fusion of all vertebrae, above and below the curve. Multiple level fixations may be used which reduce postoperative time in bed. Patient allowed up after removal of sutures. Plaster jacket or brace may be applied for extra support. Stiff curves may need anterior release followed by three weeks skeletal traction on Stryker frame prior to posterior fusion. Plaster jacket or brace applied when wounds healed. High curves need a plaster that supports under the chin and occiput. Tooth brace will be necessary to prevent dental protrusion. Treatment may continue for up to one year post-operatively.

Myogenic scoliosis. Important that patient is in bed for as little as possible. Aim is to correct spine so that patient may sit in balanced position in wheelchair. Pre-operative correction unnecessary. Dwyer anterior fusion or Luque posterior fusion performed. Very early mobilisation.

Kyphosis

Excessive posterior curvature of spine in thoracic region. Many underlying causes, e.g. Scheuermann's disease, tuberculosis of spine, osteoporosis or tumours of spine or associated with scoliosis.

Treatment. Underlying cause must be dealt with.

Lordosis

Excessive anterior curve of spine in lumbar region.
Treatment. None.

6

Conditions affecting the hips and lower limbs

THE HIPS

True hip pain is usually felt in groin and inner side of thigh. Referred hip pain felt in knee, lower spine and gluteal region.

Congenital dislocation of the hip

See Chapter 7.

Tuberculosis of the hip

Common joint to be affected. Joint erosion and abscess formation is common. Children and young adults commonly affected. 'Cold' abscess may form in gluteal muscles or thigh.

Treatment (see Chapter 1). Hip joint rested in plaster hip-spica or on traction. If cartilage or bone destroyed, joint may be arthrodesed.

Infective arthritis of hip

Not common condition but may occur in children or adolescents. Usually follows sepsis in another part of body.

Treatment (see Chapter 1). Hip usually most comfortable supported on traction until infection settles. Active physiotherapy to restore movement. If infection has destroyed joint, arthrodesis or arthroplasty may be necessary.

Rheumatoid arthritis of hip

Being larger joint not always affected by rheumatoid arthritis. If hip is affected usually gives rise to secondary osteoarthritis of hip.

Treatment (see Chapter 1). Intra-articular injections of cortisone may give temporary relief. Total hip replacement performed if joint surfaces badly destroyed.

Osteoarthritis of hip

Very common condition in elderly, or in younger persons following surgery or trauma. Pain felt in groin and thigh and referred to back and knee. Worsens on exercise, improves with rest, stiffness increases over period of time. Abduction, adduction and rotation of hip are lost first; good flexion may be maintained.

Treatment. See Chapter 1 for conservative treatments. Many operations may be performed, main ones being:

(a) Displacement osteotomy: for early osteoarthritis. Provides change of weight-bearing surfaces and weight-bearing angle through the joint. May be followed by further surgery if necessary as joint not involved.

(b) Arthroplasty: insertion of partial or total artificial joint. Partial replacement, e.g. Thompson or Austen-Moore prosthesis, used more commonly following fractured neck of femur. Femoral head only is replaced. Total replacement is common and very successful operation. Femoral component made of metal; acetabular component may be metal or plastic. The two together form a sound painfree joint (see Chapter 1). After years of use one component may loosen. Problem diagnosed by arthrography. Possible to replace faulty part. Longer bedrest post-operatively may be necessary, sometimes on traction.

(c) Excision arthroplasty (Girdlestone's operation): may be used following failed total replacement, e.g. due to infection, metal rejection or recurrent dislocation. Very successful operation for chairbound person with fixed flexion deformity of hips. By removing head of femur, shaping acetabulum and filling gap with soft muscle tissue, creates pain-free but unstable joint. Stick required for support.

(d) Arthrodesis: favoured in younger persons if other hip and knees are sound. Hip fused in about 20° flexion.

Perthes' disease

See Chapter 7.

Slipped upper femoral epiphysis

See Chapter 7.

Coxa vara

Condition in which neck-shaft angle of femur is less than normal 120°. May be congenital or following surgery, e.g. slipped upper femoral epiphysis, malunited fractures of trochanteric region of femur or metabolic conditions.

Treatment. Depends on cause. If deformity severe or disabling, corrected by femoral osteotomy (Fig. 6.1).

Coxa valga

Neck-shaft angle of femur is increased. Uncommon condition but may occur after maltreated congenital dislocation of hip.

Treatment. Displacement osteotomy of femur.

THE THIGH

Acute osteomyelitis

Femur is prone to infection. Entry through bloodstream com-

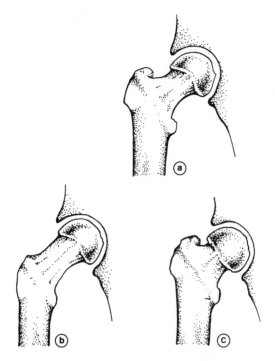

Fig. 6.1 (a) Normal neck of femur, (b) Coxa valga, (c) Coxa vara.

mon in children, or through compound wounds in adults. If lower part of femur involved, may cause effusion into knee joint.

Treatment (see Chapter 1). Neglected or maltreated acute osteomyelitis may become chronic.

Benign tumours of thigh

Giant cell tumour: osteoclastoma is commonest at lower end of femur. Invades distal end causing cortex to thin.

Treatment. Difficult to remove without disturbing knee joint. Curetted out and packed with bone chips. May recur and can become malignant.

Malignant tumours of thigh

Femur is common site for malignant tumours (see Chapter 1).

(*a*) *Osteosarcoma:* highly malignant tumour of children or young adults.

Treatment. Prophylactic treatment with cytotoxic drugs. Scans to exclude metastases. Specially made arthroplasties may be inserted. If tumour recurs, amputation may be necessary together with further cytotoxic therapy. Metastases common.

(*b*) *Metastatic tumours:* occur frequently in femur following primary tumours in breast, prostate, kidney, lung and thyroid. Pathological fractures are common.

Treatment. Primary tumours diagnosed with aid of scans. Appropriate cytotoxic therapy and/or radiotherapy may be of use. Pathological fractures fixed internally.

(*c*) *Myelamatosis* (see Chapter 1): femur is common site for tumours to settle in red bone marrow.

(*d*) *Ewing's tumour:* highly malignant tumour in children arising from the marrow. Occurs in long bones. Has 'onion-skin' appearance on X-ray due to formation of new layers of bone on top of tumour.

Treatment. Chemotherapy, radiotherapy, suitable joint replacement or amputation. Tumour metastasises rapidly causing early death.

THE KNEE

The knee is very important joint and vulnerable to injury and disease.

Tuberculosis of knee

Commonly affected joint. Very painful due to swelling and tension within joint.

Treatment (see Chapter 1). Rest and splintage essential while disease active. Exercises commenced as soon as possible. If joint surfaces damaged beyond recovery, knee arthrodesed to give pain-free joint.

Infective arthritis of knee

Knee joint frequently infected either from injury or secondary to osteomyelitis.

Treatment (see Chapter 1). Limb supported in plaster or on Thomas's splint. Traction may help severe pain. Active exercises begun as soon as infection settles.

Rheumatoid arthritis of knee

Knees are quite commonly affected by rheumatoid arthritis, usually both are involved. Painful condition, often gives rise to secondary osteoarthritis.

Treatment (see Chapter 1). During acute inflammatory stage, rest and temporary immobilisation required. Exercises begun as soon as possible. Hydrocortisone injections into joint may help temporarily.

Surgically – Synovectomy (removal of synovial membrane) may hinder joint destruction, lessen pain and increase movement. Arthroplasty with partial or total knee replacements becoming increasingly popular. Arthrodesis of knee reliable operation providing other leg can take the strain.

Osteoarthritis of knee

Commonest joint to be affected by osteoarthritis. Person is

often overweight. Past trauma, surgery or disease (e.g. rheumatoid arthritis) all predispose to osteoarthritis. Painful condition made worse by exercise. There may be effusion into joint.

Treatment (see Chapter 1). Conservative treatment tried first. Active physiotherapy to improve quadriceps to strengthen knees. Osteophytes may form loose bodies and cause joint to lock requiring removal. Some operations which may help are:

(a) Osteotomy of femur or tibia or double osteotomy of femur and tibia (Benjamin's operation) alter weight-bearing surfaces and angle through the joint.

(b) Arthroplasty: total hinged knee joint replacements becoming increasingly successful. Partial arthroplasty (e.g. McIntosh) may also be used.

(c) Arthrodesis: reliable operation if second knee is in good condition. Knee fused in 20° flexion.

Osteochondritis dissecans of knee

Commonest site of disease. Necrosis of part of articular cartilage causes bone fragments to separate forming loose bodies inside joint. May be due to damaged blood supply or injury.

Treatment. Support and rest for knee in early stages. Removal of loose body when separated from cartilage. Very prone to secondary osteoarthritis.

Chondromalacia of the patella

Affects adolescents and young adults. Articular surface of patella is roughened and causes pain on movement. Cause is unknown but condition predisposes to osteoarthritis in later life.

Treatment. Conservative treatment with crepe or elastic support. If symptoms very severe, patella may be removed.

Loose bodies in the knee

Common place for formation of loose bodies. May be due to osteochondritis dissecans, osteoarthritis or trauma.

Treatment. Removal if causing symptoms of locking within knee joint.

Recurrent dislocation of patella

Patella dislocates laterally. May be due to congenital anomaly, joint laxity of genu valgum. Affects adolescent girls more commonly than boys. May affect both knees. Patients often learn to reduce dislocation themselves.

Treatment. Physiotherapy tried first to strengthen quadriceps. Surgery may be required: patellar tendon transposed medially and reinserted into tibia to prevent further dislocation.

Tears of menisci in knees

Tears of menisci (semilunar cartilages) common especially in young men and athletes. Medial meniscus torn more commonly than lateral. Tears always occur longitudinally, may be complete through length (bucket handle tear) or torn at one end forming loose tag. Usually occurs following twisting injury, patient complains of 'locking in knee' – inability to fully extend knee.

Treatment. 'Locked knee' may require manipulation under anaesthetic to aid patient while awaiting surgery. Arthrography and arthroscopy used to confirm diagnosis. Torn part of meniscus removed either via arthroscope or by arthrotomy. Band of meniscus left if possible to prevent osteoarthritis in later life. Robert Jones pressure bandage applied post-operatively. Active and passive quadriceps exercises begun immediately and flexion exercises after removal of sutures.

Cysts of menisci

Cysts common in lateral meniscus. Often follow direct injury. Patient complains of pain mainly at night.

Treatment. Removal of cyst with meniscus if symptoms severe.

Rupture of quadriceps muscle

Can occur following flexion injury sometimes with fracture of patella or avulsion at tibial tubercle.

Treatment. Surgical repair of muscle. Patella may be removed if badly damaged. Active exercising begins once muscle has healed.

Osgood–Schlatter disease

See Chapter 7.

THE LOWER LEG

Acute osteomyelitis of tibia

Common site of infection which may enter from bloodstream or externally following compound fracture.

Treatment (see Chapter 1). Drainage of abscess likely.

Benign tumours of lower leg

Giant cell tumour (osteoclastoma) may form in upper tibia or fibula.

Treatment. If fibula only affected, whole bone removed. Upper end of tibia may be curetted and packed with bone chips. Removal of tumour, amputation or prosthetic replacement advised if any doubt about innocence of tumour.

Malignant tumours of lower leg

(a) *Osteosarcoma* often occurs at upper end of tibia.

Treatment. Whole body scan to eliminate metastases. Amputation common but specially designed prosthesis with femoral and tibial components may be inserted. Intensive chemotherapy at the same time.

(b) *Metastatic tumours* uncommon in lower limbs.

(c) *Myelomatosis* uncommon in lower limb due to lack of red bone marrow.

(d) *Ewing's tumour:* common site for highly malignant childhood tumour arising from the marrow. New layers of bone form on top of tumour.

Treatment. Chemotherapy and/or radiotherapy. Joint replacement occasionally possible. Amputation more usual. Prognosis poor – metastasises rapidly.

Bowing of tibia

See Chapter 7.

Inequality of leg length

See Chapter 7.

THE ANKLE

Tuberculosis of ankle

Rare site of infection.

Treatment (see Chapter 1). Arthrodesis may be necessary once disease is quiescent if joint has been destroyed.

Infective arthritis of ankle

Uncommon condition but may follow external injury.

Treatment. See Chapter 1.

Rheumatoid arthritis of ankle

Common joint to be affected, usually bilateral.

Treatment (see Chapter 1). Arthrodesis of joint may be necessary if pain very severe due to joint destruction.

Osteoarthritis of ankle

Less common in ankle than in larger joints. Usually secondary to rheumatoid arthritis, surgery, fractures or congenital anomaly.

Treatment (see Chapter 1). Pain in very severe cases relieved by arthrodesis of joint.

Tears of ligament of ankle

Follows severe inversion injury and requires immobilisation in plaster. If unrecognised, lateral ligament may fail to heal leading to recurrent subluxation of ankle.

Treatment. Physiotherapy to strengthen evertor muscles. If disabling, new lateral ligament may be formed by tendon transfer.

Rupture of tendo-achilles

See Chapter 3.

THE FOOT

Congenital talipes equinovarus and talipes calcaneovalgus

See Chapter 7.

Pes cavus

Associated with claw toes and high arch. May be congenital or due to neurological cause, e.g. poliomyelitis, spina bifida or peroneal muscular atrophy. Produces painful corns and callosities.

Treatment. Mild symptoms treated with chiropody. Severe symptoms corrected by surgery according to cause of pain; e.g. arthrodesis of toes to reduce clawing, muscle slide operation (Steindler) to reduce height of arch, or fusion of tarsal joints to increase foot stability.

Pes planus (flat foot)

Young children commonly have flat feet which correct themselves. Condition in older persons may be congenital or due to muscle weakness.

Treatment. Physiotherapy and insoles or medial wedges to shoes. In very severe cases tarsal bones may be arthrodesed to stabilise foot.

Osteochondritis of navicular (Köhler's disease)

Cause unknown: may be deficiency in blood supply or injury. Occurs in young children.

Treatment. Immobilisation for about three months in plaster of Paris.

Morton's metatarsalgia

Occurs commonly in middle-aged women. Pain in forefoot radiating to third and fourth toes caused by neuroma in cleft of those toes.

Treatment. Sponge-rubber metatarsal pad. If symptoms persist, cleft explored and neuroma removed.

Ganglion

Common harmless cyst occurring on dorsum of foot.

Treatment. Removal if painful or causing problems with shoes.

THE TOES

Hallux valgus

Bunion deformity occurring in two age groups.

(a) *Adolescent or young adult*: usually congenital deformity with extra long proximal phalanx of hallux.

Treatment. Osteototomy of first metatarsal. Plaster of Paris required for minimum of six weeks (Fig. 6.2).

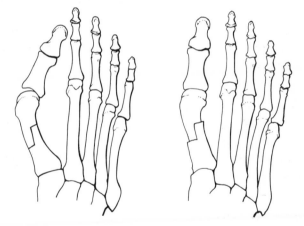

Fig. 6.2 Osteotomy of first metatarsal for juvenile hallux valgus.

(b) *Older patient*, usually middle-aged female. Painful condition. Bursa often forms over angular bunion deformity.

Treatment. Keller's operation: excision arthroplasty of metatarsophalangeal joint of hallux (Fig. 6.3) Proximal two-thirds of first phalanx excised creating pain-free fibrous joint. Exostosis and bursa also removed.

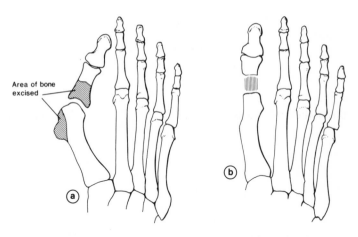

Fig. 6.3 (a) Hallux valgus deformity, (b) Keller's excision arthroplasty.

Hallux rigidus

Osteoarthritis of metatarsophalangeal joint of great toe. Causes pain on walking. Joint movements restricted.

Treatment. Adaptations to shoes, e.g. metatarsal bar to ease pressure on walking. Surgery for advanced cases: arthrodesis of metatarsophalangeal joint.

Hammer toe

Fixed deformity of interphalangeal toe joint, often second proximal interphalangeal joint. Corns may develop.

Treatment. Chiropody. Fusion of joint, e.g. peg (Fig. 6.4) or cone arthrodesis.

March fracture

See Chapter 2.

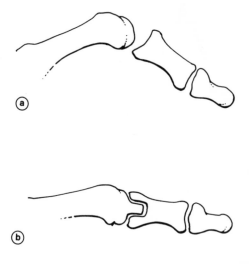

Fig. 6.4 (a) Hammer toe deformity, (b) Peg arthrodesis to fuse joint.

Osteochondritis of metatarsal head (Freiberg's disease)

Head of second or third metatarsal affected, often unilateral. Commonly affects young females. Bone head may become fragmented and deformed and lead to osteoarthritis in later life.

Treatment. In early stages bone curetted and packed with bone chips. Later stages treated symptomatically.

Ingrowing toenail

Affects great toe only. Painful and may easily become infected
Treatment. Education about cutting nails. Nail alone may be removed but will regrow. For difficult cases, nail and nail bed excised to prevent regrowth of nail.

7

Orthopaedic conditions especially related to children

Congenital deformity is one present at birth and not caused by birth injury. May be due to genetic factors, unfavourable intrauterine environment (rubella or drug taken by mother), or combination of factors.

Congenital dislocation of the hip

Very common congenital deformity, occurs four times more commonly in girls. Cause unknown. May be due to genetic and/or environmental conditions, e.g. inherited joint laxity (relaxin released in uterus from mother), and breech births. Only found in Western communities, particularly Italy and Southern France.

Hips of every child must be examined at birth and put through full range of movements. If hip dislocated or subluxed, head of femur may be felt to return to joint, sometimes with a click.

Treatment at birth. Hips require to be held in full abduction to reduce dislocation. Achieved by bulky nappies, Barlow or Von Rosen splint or rarely plaster of Paris.

If diagnosis missed at birth, not usually noticed until child starts to walk. Often late walking and may limp. If dislocation unilateral extra skin creases visible on thigh and in groin. Affected leg may 'telescope' upwards. Trendelenburg's sign is positive. Abduction of affected hip limited. Bilateral dislocations have lumbar lordosis and widening of perineum.

Later treatment. X-rays to give full detail of hips. Depending on age, closed reduction may be possible. More commonly child placed on bilateral leg traction and then legs abducted as far as possible, e.g. Burns' frame (Fig. 7.1). Adduction tenotomies may be necessary. Arthrogram performed to show outline of articular surfaces. If hip has reduced, held in frog plaster for six to nine months.

If hip not reduced, open reduction required. Various operations may be performed but aims are to increase depth of acetabulum and form roof for head of femur, to remove limbus and to reef lax limbus which prevents head of femur from entering acetabulum. Following surgery hip is held in hip spica in abduction and internal rotation. Rotation osteotomy of femoral neck required three to six weeks later to correct anteversion of femur. Hip spica immobilisation required for up to six months.

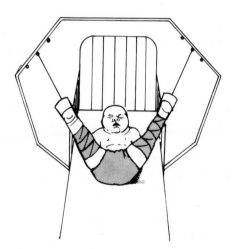

Fig. 7.1 Burn's frame. Used to gain full abduction of hips in treatment of congenital dislocation of hips.

Irritable hip

Condition often seen in young children. No definite cause found. Child limps and may complain of pain in hip or knee.

Treatment. Exclusion of Perthes' disease and other hip disorders. Rest in bed with skin traction until pain settles.

Coxa vara and coxa valga

See Chapter 6.

Slipped upper femoral epiphysis

Occurs in adolescents, more commonly in boys than girls. Child is often overweight. Presents with pain in hip and often referred to knee, limitation of hip movement and limp. Cause unknown. Lateral X-ray shows backward slip of femoral head. Bilateral slip of femoral epiphysis common, other hip must be closely watched (Fig. 72).

Treatment. Insertion of Moore or Newman pins to hold epiphysis and prevent slip from getting worse. If diagnosis has been missed and slip is severe, osteotomy of femur may be necessary. Late osteoarthritis is likely.

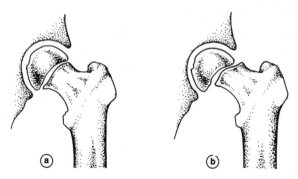

Fig. 7.2 (a) Normal hip joint, (b) slipped upper femoral epiphysis.

Congenital talipes equinovarus

Occurs in one in every thousand children, more commonly in boys. Cause unknown but may be due to intrauterine pressure. Fixed deformity noticeable at birth. Tissues on medial side of foot underdeveloped and tight. Foot is adducted, inverted and held in equinus.

Treatment. To train foot into normal shape. Treatment started 24 hours after birth. Foot is manipulated as near to correct position as possible and held with zinc oxide strapping. Manipulations repeated daily until full correction obtained. Position then held by above-knee plaster of Paris. Alternatively, Denis Browne metal splints may be used. Two splints are bolted to cross bar. Splints must be reapplied every day and checks made for sores.

If deformity will not correct conservatively or if deformity recurs, surgery required. Achilles tendon lengthened to correct equinus. Soft tissues divided on medial side of foot to release varus deformity and tendon transfers may be necessary. Foot held in plaster in position of overcorrection. Further deformity may occur as child grows. This is treated by surgery according to area of deformity.

Congenital talipes calcaneovalgus

Much less serious or common deformity. Opposite deformity to talipes equinovarus. Cause unknown. Foot held in eversion and dorsiflexion; foot almost touches shin.

Treatment. Correction started 24 hours after birth. Manual stretching by mother several times a day is usually sufficient to correct deformity. If it persists, stronger manipulation under anaesthetic may be necessary with splintage in plaster.

Osteogenesis imperfecta

Congenital inherited condition. Deficiency of osteocytes.

Sclera of eyes commonly blue. Bones extremely fragile, child may be born with multiple fractures. Further fractures frequently occur. Deformities may follow, especially bowing of long bones and spinal curvature.

Treatment. Reduction and immobilisation of fractures. Intramedullary nailing of long bones with extendable nails may be carried out to prevent deformity during growth. 'Kebab rodding' may be used for severe bowing. Legs may be protected in inflatable splints to enable child to get on to feet. Very severe cases nursed in plastazote chair and splints.

Spina bifida

Two main sections;
1. Spina bifida occulta
2. Spina bifida cystica
    (a) meningocoele
    (b) myelomeningocoele.

1. Spina bifida occulta

Malformation of vertebral arches. Meninges and spinal cord not usually affected. Tuft of hair or dimple may be visible on skin at site of defect.

2. Spina bifida cystica (Fig. 7.3)

(a) Meningocoele. Least serious of this group. Meninges only protrude through spinal gap. No major nerve involvement.

(b) Myelomeningocoele. Serious condition. Spinal cord is abnormal and protrudes into meningeal sac. Commonly found in lumbar region or at lumbar-sacral level. Often many other defects. Approximately 80% of myelomeningocoeles have

hydrocephalus – an excessive amount of cerebrospinal fluid which collects in the brain – may be due to overproduction or blockage. May develop after closure of myelomeningocoele. Hydrocephalus treated by insertion of shunt – excess cerebrospinal fluid is 'shunted' either to heart or to peritoneal cavity. Commonest valves are Spitz-Holter or Pudenz. Drainage reduces pressure.

There is paralysis of all muscles which receive nerve supply from below level of lesion. Majority of children are doubly incontinent. May have other congenital deformities: e.g. congenital dislocation of hip, fixed deformities of legs and feet or malformations of vertebrae resulting in scoliosis or kyphosis. Other deformities may develop due to muscular imbalance.

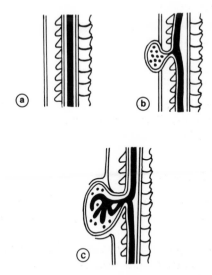

Fig. 7.3 Spina bifida (a) Cross section through normal spine, (b) Meningocoele, (c) Myelomeningocoele.

Nursing problems

1. Skin. Lack of sensation below level of lesion. Pressure sores will develop very quickly if chair seats and bony prominences not padded. Frequent change of position essential. Heat and cold cannot be felt. Precautions taken to avoid burns and exposure to cold.

2. Incontinence. Lack of urinary sphincter control. Dribbling incontinence. No bladder sensation. Renal reflux, hydronephrosis and recurrent infection present many problems. Bladder may be controlled by manual expression, appliances or intermittent catheterisation. Many have urinary diversion. Bowels – total lack of sphincter control. No sensation of need to defaecate. Chronic constipation is common. Necessary to develop pattern of bowel habits, maybe laxatives, suppositories or manual evacuation.

Orthopaedic problems

Fixed deformities may occur at joints, requiring muscle and tendon releases and joint arthrodeses when growth complete. Scoliosis often occurs, necessitating correction and fusion often in two stages to allow child to sit in chair in straight position. Other congenital deformities: e.g. dislocated hips and talipes equinovarus are common and require treatment.

Muscular disorders

There are numerous disorders, many of which are congenital. Diagnosis may be made by muscle biopsy. Weakness in muscles can produce deformity, usually due to imbalance.

Duchenne muscular dystrophy

The worst and most progressive muscular disorder. Occurs

in 2.5 of every 10 000 boys. Usually noticed when child first starts to walk. Falls and is frequently clumsy in all movements. Incurable condition at present. Condition worsens through early childhood and may require wheelchair by the time they are teenagers and sometimes before. Prognosis is very poor and majority die in late teens from respiratory and cardiac complications.

Many develop scoliosis due to muscular imbalance which makes sitting in chair difficult and uncomfortable. Bent position leads to deformity of chest, accelerating death. Posterior fusion of spine – e.g. Luque or multiple level Harrington fixation – may be carried out. Very early mobilisation essential to prevent further deterioration of muscles due to inactivity. See Chapter 5.

Cerebral palsy

Spastic paralysis due to brain damage before, during, or after birth. May be spastic type or athetoid (continuous uncontrolled movements). Intelligence, any of the senses, and emotional control may be affected. Any one or more or all four limbs may be affected. Orthopaedic conditions arise due to fixed deformities at joints, e.g. equinus deformity at ankle corrected by elongation of Achilles tendon, adduction of hips corrected by tenotomies. Arthrodesis of joints useful when bone growth complete.

Infantile torticollis

Condition arises between birth and six months. Tight sternomastoid muscle causes deformity: lateral flexion of affected side, chin points to opposite foot.

Treatment. In early stages muscle can be stretched by physiotherapy. In established cases surgery required to divide muscle. Physiotherapy needed once wound is healed.

Sprengel's shoulder

Congenital elevation of scapula. May be associated with scoliosis. Range of shoulder movement limited but disability usually minimal.

Treatment. Usually nothing but surgery may be attempted if cosmetic correction wanted. Muscles attached to lower portion of scapula and upper portion excised.

Congenital and infantile idiopathic scoliosis

See Chapter 6

Inequality of leg length

Cause of short leg may be:

(a) Congenital dislocated hip, coxa vara, idiopathic achondroplasia.

(b) Inflammatory: septic arthritis, osteomyelitis, anterior poliomyelitis.

(c) Traumatic: malunion of fractures, non-reductions of dislocations.

Long leg may be due to:

(a) Neurofibroma.

(b) Arteriovenous fistula: increase in blood supply gives extra growth.

Treatment. If discrepancy is 1.3 cm or less, best forgotten. Shoe raise used for greater differences.

Leg lengthening

May be carried out on femur or tibia or both before epiphyses fused. Two inches may be gained on each bone. Wagner apparatus commonly used. Bone drilled to weaken it and then fractured with little damage to periosteum (Fig. 7.4). Appar-

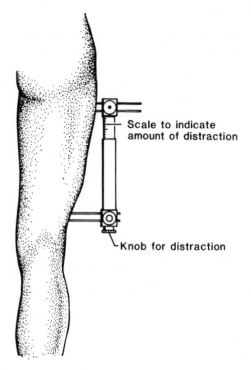

**Scale to indicate
amount of distraction**

Knob for distraction

Fig. 7.4 Wagner apparatus for leg lengthening.

atus distracted daily – child may be taught to do it under
supervision. When full length obtained, plate attached by
screws over gap. Apparatus removed (Fig. 7.5). Additional
bone graft may be added at this time. Nursed in slings and
springs traction for up to six weeks. Important to watch for
overstretching of nerves during distraction. May be seen as
pain or patches of numbness. Essential to keep knee and hip
fully mobile during lengthening. Attention to pins to prevent
infection.

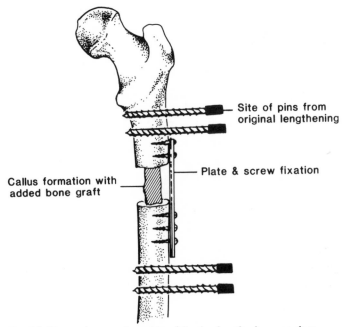

Site of pins from original lengthening

Plate & screw fixation

Callus formation with added bone graft

Fig. 7.5 Plate and screws in position following lengthening procedure.

Leg shortening

If person tall and can afford to lose height, legs equalised by shortening the longer one. Growth may be slowed in a bone by epiphysiodesis (destroying epiphysis) or stapling epiphysis. Femur may be shortened by removing appropriate amount of bone, usually from below lesser trochanter. Held with pin and plate fixation.

Genu valgum (knock knees) (Fig. 7.6)

Commonly seen in young children when cause unknown. May also be due to endocrine disease or rickets.

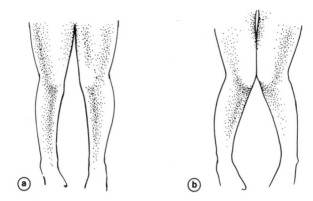

Fig. 7.6 (a) Genu varum. (b) Genu valgum.

Treatment. Idiopathic condition commonly corrects itself with growth. If condition progressive, medial femoral staples fixed to retard growth. May be removed when growth equal.

Genu varum (bow legs)

Commonly seen in toddlers. Important to exclude underlying bone disease.

Treatment. Usually none. If condition persists corrective osteotomy may be necessary.

Genu recurvatum

Hyperextension deformity of knee. Uncommon. May be congenital or following paralysis, e.g. anterior poliomyelitis.

Treatment. Usually none. Paralytic patient controls knee and creates deformity with muscle power. Tibial osteotomy may help congenital cosmetic deformity.

Osteochondritis juvenilis

Condition affecting growing epiphysis or ossifying small bone in child. Cause unknown. Avascular necrosis may occur. New blood vessels grow into bone again and revascularise area. Complete recovery may be possible. Same condition in different bones has different names.

(a) *Perthes' disease*: osteochondritis of epiphysis of femoral head. Interruption of blood supply to femoral head resulting in avascular necrosis. Reason unknown. Femoral head becomes softened and may flatten and become deformed. Predisposes to osteoarthritis in later life. Occurs in 5–10 year olds, more commonly in boys. Often first noted as limp. Pain may be referred to knee.

Treatment. Protection of hip to prevent further deformity. May take up to four years for femoral head to reform. Rotational osteotomy prevents severe damage of head and allows early mobilisation. Long-term conservative use of caliper may sometimes be adopted.

(b) *Scheuermann's disease*: osteochondritis of spine. (See Chapter 5).

(c) *Osgood-Schlatter disease*: pain and swelling over tibial tubercle. Not always classified as osteochondritis. X-ray may show fragmentation.

Treatment. Restriction of activity until pain settles. Plaster cylinder if pain acute.

(d) *Freiburg's disease*: osteochondritis of head of second metatarsal (see Chapter 6).

(e) *Keinbock's disease*: osteochondritis of lunate (see Chapter 4).

Rickets

Metabolic disorder. In adults known as osteomalacia. May be due to deficiency of vitamin D, resistance to vitamin D or renal rickets.

(a) *Vitamin D deficiency*: vitamin D is essential for absorption of calcium necessary for bone production. Normally obtained from diet and sunlight. Lack of calcium in children softens developing bones causing curvatures of long bones and swellings of epiphyses.

Treatment. Oral vitamin D (calciferol). Early nutritional rickets responds well. Established bowing of tibiae may require osteotomy.

(b) *Vitamin D resistant*: inherited condition. Symptoms as before but seen in younger child.

Treatment. Very large doses of vitamin D.

(c) *Renal rickets*: congenital or acquired kidney damage. Phosphorous retained in blood and prevents absorption of calcium. Deformities may be severe and child dwarfed and ill looking.

Treatment. To correct kidney condition if possible. Diet supplemented with vitamin D and calcium. Bony deformities corrected surgically if necessary.

Still's disease

Juvenile rheumatoid arthritis (see Chapter 8).

8

Rheumatological conditions

RHEUMATOID ARTHRITIS

Chronic systemic disease of unknown cause. Three times more common in women, usually affecting those 25–40 years old. Onset is usually gradual; disease runs progressive course with periods of remission. Small joints, fingers, toes, wrists and ankles, affected first.

Pathology

1. Synovial membrane is inflamed causing swelling of joint, capsule and tissues, effusion into joint and thinning of adjacent bone cortex and trabeculae (Fig. 8.1b). All result in acute pain and stiffness.

2. Inflamed synovial membrane thickens and actively destroys nearby structures. Articular cartilage thins and is replaced by pannus (Fig. 8.1c). Synovial membrane penetrates into bone not protected by articular cartilage and gradually destroys it. Ligaments attacked from within joint.

3. During normal use of joint or after stress, ligaments and tendons stretch and tear. Bone collapses and crumbles where undermined (Fig. 8.1d). Articular cartilage thinned and roughened and subject to secondary osteoarthritis. Growing synovium fills joint space and can get wedged. Joint unstable and deformed because of collapsed bone, thin articular cartilage, stretched weakened ligaments and tendons, weak

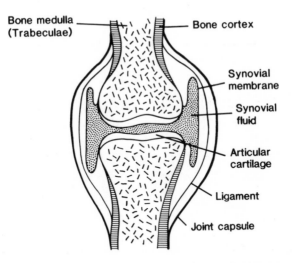

Fig. 8.1 (a) A normal joint

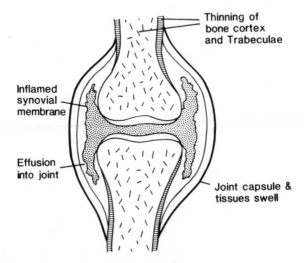

Fig. 8.1 (b) Stage 1. Joint is stiff and painful

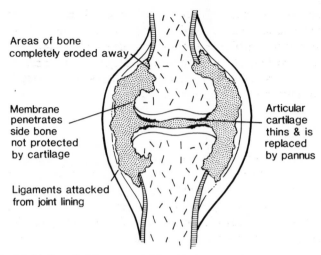

Areas of bone completely eroded away

Membrane penetrates side bone not protected by cartilage

Articular cartilage thins & is replaced by pannus

Ligaments attacked from joint lining

Fig. 8.1 (c) Stage 2. Joint very painful and becoming unstable

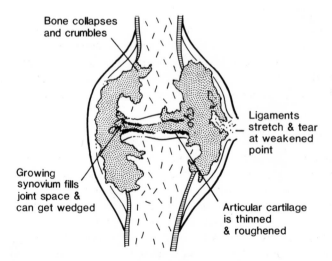

Bone collapses and crumbles

Ligaments stretch & tear at weakened point

Growing synovium fills joint space & can get wedged

Articular cartilage is thinned & roughened

Fig. 8.1 (d) Stage 3. Joint unstable and deformed. Movement limited and painful.

wasted muscles and enlarged synovium which pushes joint capsule and tendons out of line. Joint movement limited because articular cartilage rough and jagged; pain from inflamed tissues, swelling of joint by fluid and synovial membrane, weak muscles and ruptured tendons and, possibly, paralysis due to inflammation pressing on nerves.

Investigations

Blood investigations may show raised erythrocyte sedimentation rate, moderate anaemia, positive latex fixation test and positive sheep cell agglutination test (SCAT).

X-rays show swelling of soft tissues around joints, loss of bone near joints (periarticular osteoporosis), narrowing of joint space, erosion of bone and deformities of joints.

Signs and symptoms

Disease onset is usually gradual but may be acute with fever. Patient complains of pain, warmth and swelling of one or more joints particularly with early morning stiffness. Rheumatoid arthritis normally follows symmetrical pattern in body. Patient is often in poor health, anaemic and depressed.

Treatment

1. Reduce inflammation in joints; bedrest and complete rest of joints for four weeks, splints and casts as necessary.
2. Relieve pain and depression – drugs and counselling.
3. Prevent further damage to joints – change of work if necessary, power sparing gadgets and splints.
4. Synovectomy: removal of synovial lining to joint removes nerve supply to joint and therefore removes pain. May slow down joint destruction. Particularly useful in fingers and knees.

5. Further surgery may be performed to save joint:
   (a) Tendon suture and repair – for hands, wrists and fingers.
   (b) Arthroplasty: (i) total hip, knee and possibly elbow and shoulder replacements.
   (ii) silastic replacement spacers for metacarpophalangeal joints.
   (c) Excision arthroplasty – Fowler's operation to excise metatarsal heads, relieves pain in deformed foot.
   (d) Arthrodesis – cervical spine C1 on C2 when instability present. Wrist in late stages.
6. Rehabilitation (Fig. 8.2):
   (a) Sticks, crutches, wheelchairs, adapted cars, etc.,
   (b) Orthopaedic footwear.
   (c) Splints, gadgets and aids to daily living.
   (d) Visits to patient's home and adaptations to it as necessary.
   (e) Arrangements for home help, community nurse, meals on wheels, community social worker, etc., as necessary.

Drugs

Aspirin to reduce inflammation is still drug of choice for rheumatoid arthritis but frequently causes gastric irritation. Soluble and enteric-coated tablets better tolerated. Many different anti-inflammatory drugs available. These help pain but may also cause gastric disturbances. Weekly gold injections (Myocrisin) help pain in some patients but may cause kidney damage. Urine must be tested weekly for albumin. Corticosteroids used very rarely these days because of side effects but have a use in the elderly patient in severe pain. Cytotoxic drugs are sometimes used in older patient with severe disease. Not used in younger patient as can induce neoplasm.

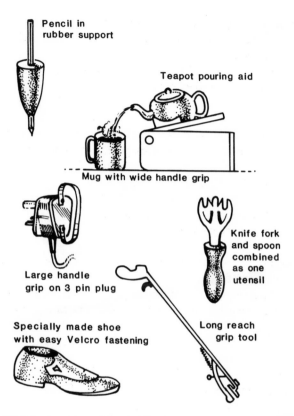

Fig. 8.2 Selective aids used in rehabilitation.

Juvenile rheumatoid arthritis

Occurs in children under 16 years of age. Two main types:

1. Still's disease

Most common in girls and often in very young children. Child has high fever and may have rash and enlargement of glands, liver and spleen. May develop pericarditis and inflammation of iris leading to permanent sight damage. Children develop acute joint pains – usually in larger joints first – e.g. knees and wrists.

2. Polyarthritis

Similar to Still's disease but smaller joints affected first, as in rheumatoid arthritis. Neck often affected. May have tenosynovitis of flexor tendons. Often have growth disturbances – e.g. leg inequality or underdeveloped jaw.

Treatment. As for adults with rheumatoid arthritis. Drug of choice is aspirin.

Gout

Inflammation of synovial membrane caused by crystals of uric acid. Commonest joint affected is metatarsophalangeal joint of hallux. Any joint may be affected. Joint is hot, swollen, red and painful. Blood test shows raised uric acid.

Treatment. Rest, analgesia and anti-inflammatory drugs. Probenecid used prophylactically to reduce level of uric acid.

Further reading

Adams J Crawford 1981 Outline of orthopaedics, 9th edn. Churchill Livingstone, Edinburgh

Adams J Crawford 1981 Outline of fractures, including joint injuries, 8th edn. Churchill Livingstone, Edinburgh

Hughes S, Sweetnam R 1980 Basis and practice of orthopaedics. Heinemann, London

McRae R K 1983 Clinical orthopaedic examination, 2nd edn. Churchill Livingstone, Edinburgh

Powell M 1982 Orthopaedic nursing and rehabilitation, 8th edn. Churchill Livingstone, Edinburgh

Pinney E 1978 Orthopaedic nursing, 6th edn. Balliere Tindall, London

Fleetcroft J P 1983 The musculo-skeletal system. Churchill Livingstone, Edinburgh

Farrell J 1982 Illustrated guide to orthopaedic nursing. Lippincott, Philadelphia

Stewart J D M, Hallett J P 1983 Traction and orthopaedic appliances, 2nd edn. Churchill Livingstone, Edinburgh

Index